INGREDIENTS OF A BALANCED DIET

Vegetables

Rachel Eugster

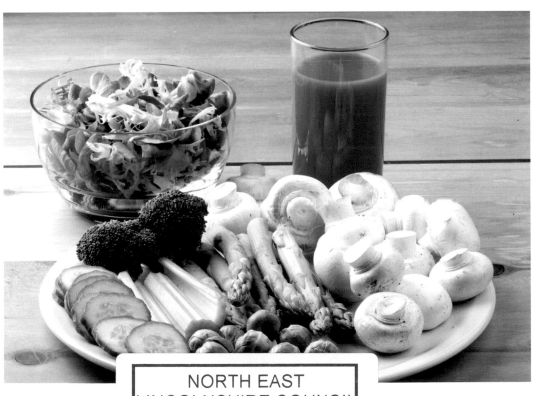

This edition 2010

Franklin Watts
338 Euston Road,
London NW1 3BH

Franklin Watts Australia
Level 17/207 Kent Street
Sydney NSW 2000

INGREDIENTS OF A BALANCED DIET:
VEGETABLES was produced for Franklin
Watts by Bender Richardson White, PO Box
266, Uxbridge, UK.
Editor and Picture Researcher: Lionel Bender
Designer and Page Make-up: Ben White
Cover Make-up: Mike Pilley, Radius
Production: Kim Richardson
Graphics and Maps: Stefan Chabluk

A CIP catalogue record for this book is
available from the British Library.

Every attempt has been made to clear
copyright. Should there be any inadvertent
omission please apply to the publisher for
rectification.

ISBN: 978 0 7496 9643 6
Dewey classification: 641.3'5

Printed in China

Franklin Watts is a division of Hachette
Children's Books, an Hachette UK company.
www.hachette.co.uk

Picture credits

Cover image: FoodandDrinks agency.
foodanddrinkphotos.com: pages 1, 5, 8, 11, 20, 27
top. iStockphotos: pages 1, 3, 30, 31, 32 and all
Food bite panels (Sergey Kashkin); pages 3 and 15
(Ursula Alter); page 3 and all Recipe boxes
(Amanda Rohde); pages 4 (Ivan Scott); 6 (Lisa
Gagne); 7 (Chris Bence); 9 (Georgios Alexandris);
10 (Sawomire Fajer); 12; 14 (Julian Pond); 15
(Wojciech Krusinski); 16; 17 (Kelly Cline); 18
(Carmen Martinez Banús); 19 (Daniel St. Pierre);
21 (Luc Gillet); 22 (Matthew Cole); 25; 26 (Sheri
Bigelow); 27b (Carmen Martinez Banús); 29 top
(Tina Rencelj); 29 bottom (Sara Labrooy).
Cover image: foodanddrinkphotos.com.
BRW wishes to thank Sarah Bell and colleagues at
foodanddrinkphotos.com for setting up the
commissioned photography.

The author

Rachel Eugster is a food, health and
nutrition writer and editor. Formerly food
editor of *Walking* magazine, she is a
regular contributor to *Continental* and
YES Mag and creates recipes for people of
all ages. She feeds her family as healthy a
diet as they will eat!

The consultant

Ester Davies is a professional food and
nutrition writer, lecturer and consultant.
She has a B.Ed. in Food, Nutrition and
Sociology. She has written books on food
specifically for the National Curriculum.

Note: In recipes, liquid measures and
small quantities are given by volume in
millilitres (ml) as this is how measuring
jugs and spoons are usually marked.

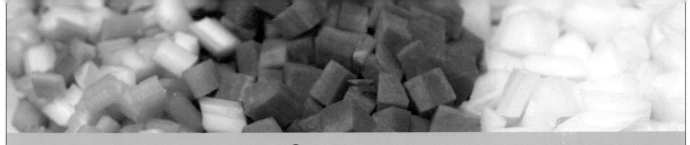

Contents

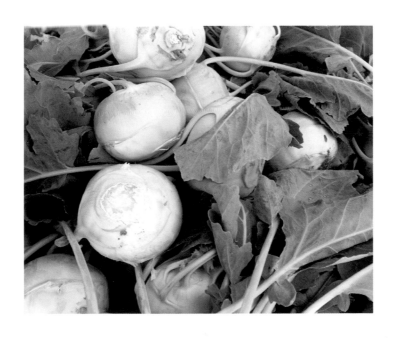

Major nutrients

Vegetables, like other foods, contain a mix of nutrients. The following are the most important.

Sugars and starches, or carbohydrates: give you energy. Fibre is a kind of carbohydrate that aids digestion.

Proteins: provide building materials for bones, hair, muscles and skin.

Vitamins and minerals: help you fight diseases and digest food, and strengthen your bones and teeth.

Fats: store energy for later use and carry vitamins to where they are needed. Unsaturated fat (from plant foods) is better for you than saturated fat (from meat and dairy foods).

Introducing vegetables

A vegetable is any part of a plant that is used for food. There are many kinds of vegetables. Carrots and parsnips, for example, are root vegetables. Celery and rhubarb are stem vegetables. When we eat asparagus and cabbages, we are eating the entire plants except for their roots. Potatoes are tubers, which are swollen, underground stems from which new plants can grow.

We also eat the leaves, buds, flowers, seeds, fruits and bulbs of plants. Mushrooms and seaweeds are eaten as vegetables, too. There are hundreds of kinds and varieties of vegetables eaten around the world.

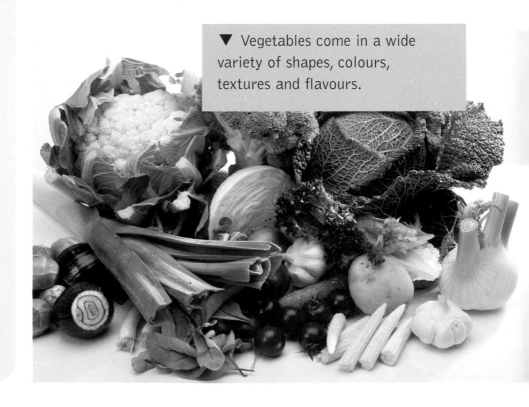

▼ Vegetables come in a wide variety of shapes, colours, textures and flavours.

Good for your body

Vegetables are rich in minerals, vitamins and fibre. They also contain some proteins and carbohydrates. These are the main nutrients your body needs in varying amounts but cannot make itself. You need a special mix of nutrients for growth and to keep you fit and healthy. In addition to nutrients, vegetables contain some of the energy that your body needs to stay active (see pages 24–25).

A balanced diet

'Balancing' your diet means eating and drinking just the right amounts and types of healthy foods and avoiding unhealthy foods, particularly those rich in sugars and saturated fats. You should eat at least five servings of vegetables and fruits a day. A serving can be a glass of tomato or carrot juice, a half a cupful of cooked broccoli, carrots or peas, or a small bowl of green salad such as lettuce, peppers and celery.

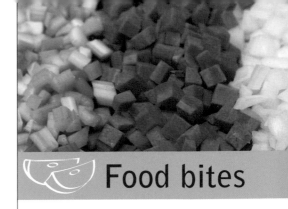

Fruits, pulses and bulbs

Many vegetables are actually fruits, which are the parts of plants that produce seeds. They include tomatoes, cucumbers, pumpkins, aubergines and red and green peppers.

The pods of beans, peas and lentils are also fruits. Sometimes, we eat the complete pods as vegetables, as with runner beans and mangetout. Sometimes we eat just the seeds, as with broad beans and green peas. When dried, beans, peas and lentils are usually known as pulses.

New plants grow not just from seeds but also from bulbs. Onions, swedes and fennel are examples of bulbs eaten as vegetables.

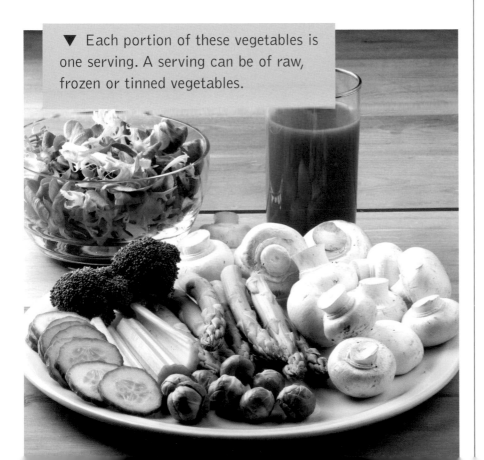

▼ Each portion of these vegetables is one serving. A serving can be of raw, frozen or tinned vegetables.

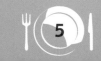

To go with vegetables

What kinds of dishes and meals can you make with vegetables for a balanced diet? To help you decide, dieticians have created the idea of food groups, like those listed to the right. You should eat more from groups at the top of the list and less of those at the bottom of the list.

You can eat vegetables with red meat, such as beef and lamb. Poultry, or white meat, for example turkey and chicken, goes well with most vegetables. Eat poultry without the skin on and not fried. Fish is a great alternative to poultry, but again you should not eat it fried. Eggs and low-fat dairy products – cheese and yogurt – are good with vegetables, too. At all times, avoid eating a lot of fatty or sugary foods.

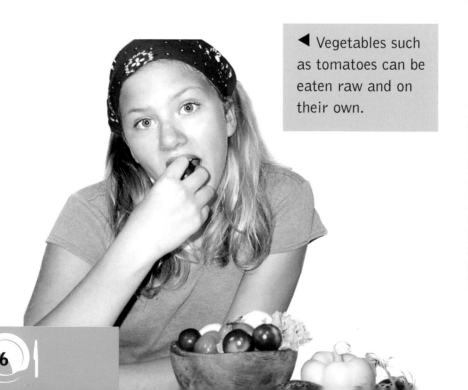

◄ Vegetables such as tomatoes can be eaten raw and on their own.

Nutrition facts

Food groups

Most dieticians group foods into five categories according to the mix of nutrients they contain.

1. **Bread and other grain products, and potatoes.** These are rich in carbohydrates (including fibre), proteins, minerals and vitamins.
2. **Fruits and vegetables.** Both are rich in carbohydrates (including fibre), vitamins and minerals.
3. **Milk and dairy products.** They are rich in calcium and proteins.
4. **Meat, fish, eggs, nuts, seeds and pulses.** These are good sources of proteins, minerals and B vitamins.
5. **Fatty, sugary and salty foods.** These can have some good nutrients but are high in calories, salt and saturated fats.

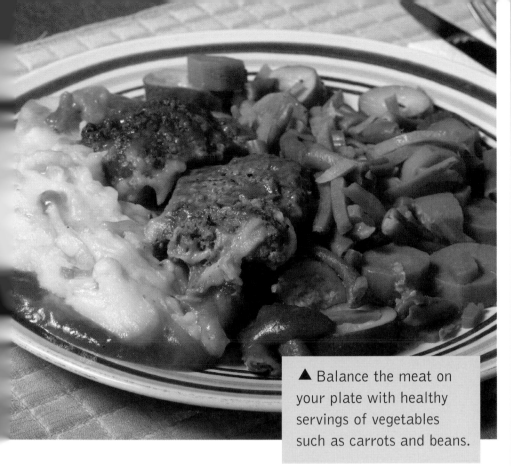

▲ Balance the meat on your plate with healthy servings of vegetables such as carrots and beans.

The three-quarter rule

One way to build a balanced diet is to imagine that your plate is divided into four equal sections. Fill one quarter with protein-rich foods such as red meat, poultry, dairy products, fish, nuts or pulses. Fill the other three quarters with other foods. These can be vegetables, brown rice, potatoes, bread or pasta – any food from the first and second food groups. This small change can make a big difference in your diet.

A meatless diet

If you are a vegetarian – a person who does not eat meat – you can make vegetables a major part of your diet. You must, though, eat a variety of vegetables along with whole grains, pulses, nuts, dairy foods and fruit. This way you will get all the nutrients and energy you need (see pages 20–21). Vegans – people who do not eat any animal foods – leave out dairy foods.

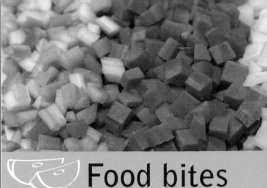

Food bites

Non-plant vegetables

Mushrooms are fungi and seaweeds are algae. They do not grow from seeds or bulbs. Instead, they grow from tiny spores. Mushrooms are eaten raw in salads or cooked and used in soups, stews, casseroles, pizzas, omelettes and vegetable dishes. Seaweeds are eaten in soups and salads or wrapped round fish.

Mushrooms are full of proteins, B vitamins and minerals such as potassium. There are 38,000 varieties of mushroom, some of which are edible and others poisonous. The most popular edible varieties include white button, chanterelle, crimini, morel, porcini and portabello.

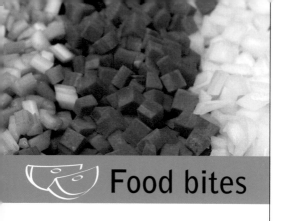

Water in food

You drink only half the water you need. The rest comes from your food. Vegetables contain a high percentage of water compared to other foods:

celery: 95%
potatoes, raw: 78%
potatoes, boiled: 81%
mushrooms: 92%
lettuce: 96%
kidney beans: 77%
haricot beans: 11%
cabbage, raw: 88%
cabbage, boiled: 93%
onions: 93%
watercress 91%

▶A mix of raw, colourful peppers and varieties of lettuce makes a vegetable side-dish suitable for almost any meal.

More about nutrients

Vegetables can provide more than 20% of the water you need, 50% of the vitamin C and 25% of the vitamin A (see page 23). Their low energy and high fibre content means you can eat lots of them and feel full without putting on weight.

Vitamins and minerals

Leafy vegetables tend to be rich in vitamin C, calcium, iron and fibre. Root vegetables, tubers and bulbs are good sources of carbohydrates and fibre. Some vegetables are especially rich in certain vitamins and minerals. Asparagus has lots of folic acid and vitamin C, carrots are rich in vitamin A, and chicory is a good source of calcium, magnesium and B vitamins.

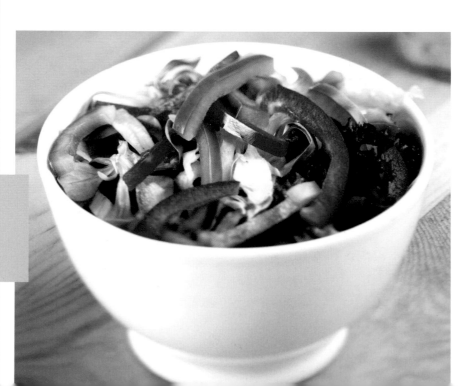

Nutrition facts

Fibre in vegetables

Vegetables contain lots of fibre, or roughage, which helps you digest food and pass it through your digestive system. Fibre also lowers the amount of cholesterol in your bloodstream. Cholesterol is a chemical made by the body. High levels of cholesterol in your body can lead to heart disease.

Low on bad things

Fresh vegetables contain very little of the things you should avoid – saturated fat, salt and refined sugar. Saturated fat is the source of cholesterol. Too much salt raises your blood pressure. Refined sugar has high levels of energy and is bad for your teeth.

Vegetables are also a source of phytochemicals, which are substances in food that work together to keep you healthy. They are also high in antioxidants, which are substances that prevent cell damage.

Effects on nutrients

The nutrient content of vegetables varies depending on the variety, how and where they are grown, when they are harvested, in what way and for how long they are stored and how they are cooked. Remember this when you look at tables and charts of nutrients in food and on food labels in shops.

Vitamin C is destroyed by sunlight so vegetables on an outdoor market stall may have lost some goodness. Peeling vegetables removes some nutrients, but also pesticides and dirt. Vitamin C and vitamin B1 are largely destroyed by heat. When vegetables are boiled in water, some of the minerals are washed out.

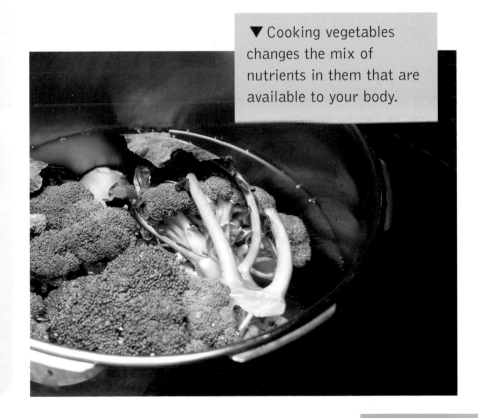

▼ Cooking vegetables changes the mix of nutrients in them that are available to your body.

Choice of vegetables

Some people choose vegetables based on cost. Produce grown locally is usually easier and cheaper to buy than produce grown far away.

The climate where you live and the seasons can also influence what is available in your shops. In many places, for example, fresh vegetables are more plentiful in the summer and autumn.

Families from different countries may have been brought up eating different vegetables from you. They will be used to different flavours and mixes of food. Discuss with your friends the vegetables you like and why.

New ideas

You can eat vegetables in many ways. Lettuce, carrots, celery, radishes, tomatoes and peppers can all be eaten raw, on their own, in salads or in sandwiches. Many vegetables can be eaten in pies, flans, casseroles, soups, burgers, pizzas and sausages. Others, such as cooked broccoli, cauliflower, Brussels sprouts, potatoes, swedes, parsnips, turnips and cabbage, go well with red meat and poultry dishes.

Below average

Many people eat only three servings of vegetables and fruits a day. Potatoes do not count as a serving as they are mostly carbohydrates – but they do contain minerals and vitamins. To improve your diet, look for new ways to eat vegetables. Try vegetable juices such as carrot, red pepper, parsnip and tomato. If you find their taste unusual, try adding a little flavour to them, such as Worcester sauce.

▼ Adding lettuce and tomato to a sandwich is one way to eat vegetables. Try others, too, such as cucumber and alfalfa sprouts.

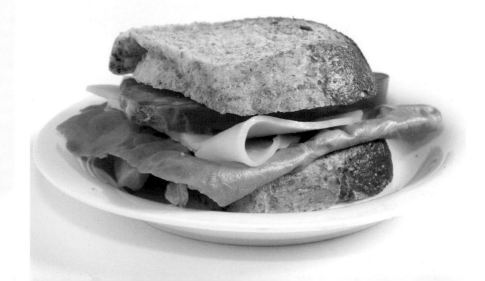

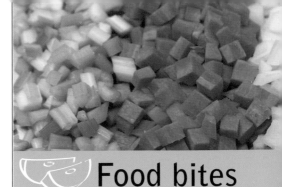

From stews to chutney and burgers

Some vegetables, such as onions, garlic and chillies, or hot peppers, have a strong taste. Others may have textures or flavours you find unusual. Try these vegetables a little at a time, or mix them into stews, casseroles or pasta.

Some vegetables can be dried, pickled or made into chutneys, and you may find these more to your taste. Pickling involves bottling food in vinegar, oil or salt water. Chutneys are made by chopping vegetables and cooking them with spices, vinegar and sugar. They can be eaten with meat and cheese, or with a curry.

Green peppers, courgettes, onions and other vegetables can be mixed with potatoes, eggs or grains and baked to make vegetable burgers. Tomato sauce or salsa can be added for extra flavour.

Vegetable snack

Next time friends or relatives come to your house for a party or sleepover, put out some dishes or bowls of raw vegetable slices. The slices will make perfect snacks.

Use baby carrots, celery, broccoli, cauliflower, radishes, fennel, cherry tomatoes and colourful pepper strips. You can also add some tasty dips such as hummus, egg mayonnaise, salsa or cream cheese. Watch to see how quickly your friends eat the vegetables.

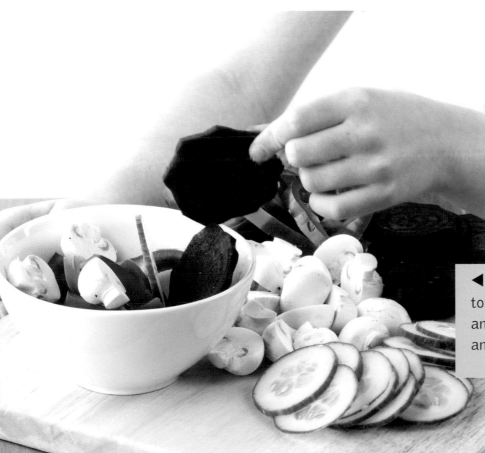

◀ Vegetables such as cucumber, tomatoes, peppers, mushrooms and beetroot can be easily cut up and made into a salad.

An amazing variety

For many vegetables eaten around the world, there are several varieties. Each variety may have a different colour, texture and flavour from the main type. Also, each vegetable may have various names around the world. For example, aubergines are also called eggplants, okra is lady's fingers and squash is often known as marrow but is a separate vegetable, too.

Vegetable groups

Vegetables are grouped in many ways. As mentioned on pages 5 and 6, they can be grouped by the part of the plant – leaf, stem, root, and so on. The cabbage family – scientifically the *Brassica* family – includes cabbage,

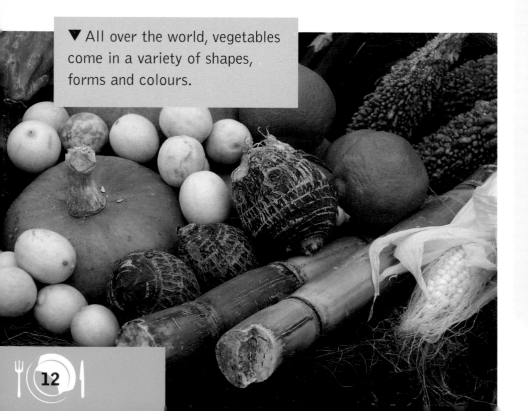

▼ All over the world, vegetables come in a variety of shapes, forms and colours.

Nutrition facts

Organic vegetables

Organic food is grown without using artificial pesticides and fertilisers. Organic farmers do not grow genetically modified (GM) foods. So should you buy and eat organic vegetables? That depends on many things.

Organic farming does less harm to the environment and organic food may look better, taste better and offer more nutrients. Sometimes, though, organic produce may be marked or bruised or look oddly shaped, and it may spoil faster. It can also be expensive.

The main thing is to eat enough fresh vegetables every day, whether they are organically grown or not.

broccoli, cauliflower, Brussels sprouts and kale. Among the leafy and salad vegetables are chickory, dandelion, endive, lettuce, mustard greens, spinach, Swiss chard and watercress. Peppers, cucumbers, aubergines, marrows and pumpkins are fruiting vegetables.

An expanding range

In earlier times, available vegetables were limited to those that grew nearby or were in season. Nowadays, vegetables are flown or shipped from faraway places to markets all over the world.

Vegetables that were once known only where they grow, such as Jerusalem artichoke from North America, endives from Asia and okra from Africa, are now more readily available. New varieties of vegetables are being introduced all the time, gradually becoming popular internationally.

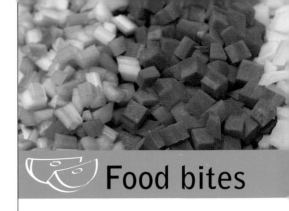

Food bites

High costs

Transporting vegetables around the world uses up costly fuels and increases pollution from vehicles. Also, some of the vegetables' nutrients are lost between harvesting and getting them to the kitchen table.

Where in the world?

The red dots on the map shows where some exotic vegetables are produced in large amounts. How many of the named vegetables are you familiar with? See if you can find out more about them. Most of them can be grown in a variety of climates.

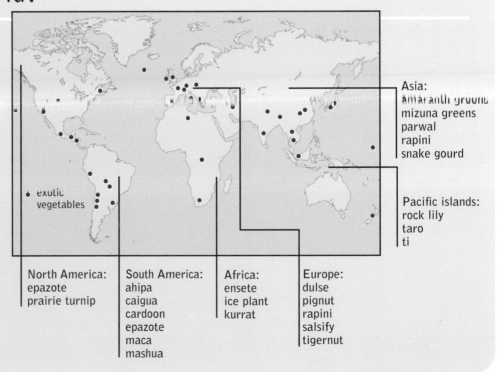

exotic vegetables

Asia:
amaranth greens
mizuna greens
parwal
rapini
snake gourd

Pacific islands:
rock lily
taro
ti

North America:
epazote
prairie turnip

South America:
ahipa
caigua
cardoon
epazote
maca
mashua

Africa:
ensete
ice plant
kurrat

Europe:
dulse
pignut
rapini
salsify
tigernut

Vegetable colours

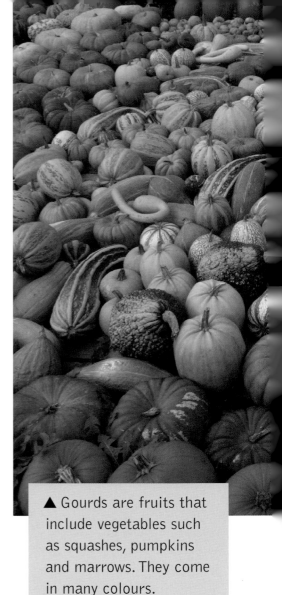

▲ Gourds are fruits that include vegetables such as squashes, pumpkins and marrows. They come in many colours.

C hoose vegetables of as many different colours as you can. This will give you the best mix of nutrients. Vegetables can be white or red, orange, yellow, green or purple – all the colours of the rainbow.

Colour code

Each colour of vegetable is associated with its own set of phytochemicals and antioxidants – nutrients that work together to protect your health. In most cases, the more deeply coloured the vegetable, the more of these nutrients it is likely to have. Orange vegetables (carrots, most sweet potatoes and pumpkins) and dark green vegetables (collards or kales, broccoli and watercress) are particularly rich in these nutrients.

Nutrition facts

colour	health benefits	examples
green	healthy eyes; prevents cancer	kale, chard, Brussels sprouts, spinach
yellow-orange	healthy heart and immune system; prevents cancer	carrots, some sweet potatoes, marrows, pumpkins, butternut squash, sweetcorn
red	fights diabetes, high blood pressure and cancers	red cabbage, red pepper, beets, radishes, rhubarb, tomatoes
purple	prevents cancer and heart disease	aubergines, kohlrabis, radishes, onions
white	healthy heart; prevents cancer	garlic, onions, leeks, shallots

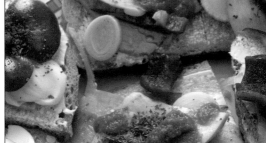

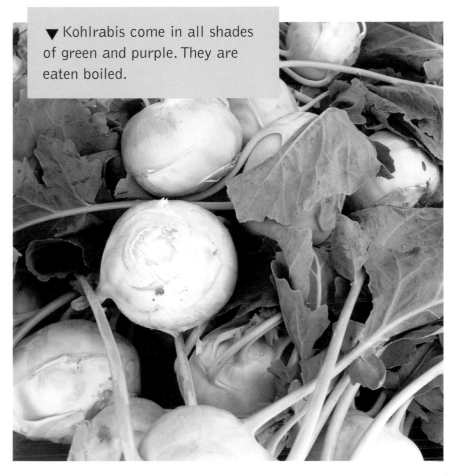

▼ Kohlrabis come in all shades of green and purple. They are eaten boiled.

New colours

Nowadays, you can buy familiar vegetables in unexpected new colours. Some are traditional varieties that fell out of fashion but are being reintroduced, such as brown sweet peppers. Other varieties have been newly developed by plant-growers and farmers. For example, carrots now come not just in orange and purple but also in red, yellow, green, white or black. Purple potatoes, asparagus, endive and peppers are also available.

Yellow beets, orange cauliflower and red sweetcorn offer a package of phytochemicals and antioxidants that is different from that of their traditional varieties. Not only do these new colours look intriguing and make dishes more attractive, but they are also good for you.

Recipe

Vegetable frittatas

Makes 8 servings.
Ingredients
125g mushrooms, chopped
1 400-g tin artichoke hearts, drained
1 plum tomato, chopped
1/2 green pepper, chopped
200g cooked spinach, chopped
125g cheddar cheese, grated
10 eggs
5ml oregano
5ml basil
2.5ml rosemary
pepper, to taste

Preparation
Preheat the oven to 180°C (Gas mark 4). Grease a baking dish or an oven-proof frying pan.
Mix the vegetables together and spread them in the dish or pan. Cover with the cheese.
In a bowl, beat the eggs with the herbs and pepper. Pour this over the vegetables.
Bake for about 40 minutes or until the eggs are set. The frittata can be eaten hot or cold, as a snack or a light main course.

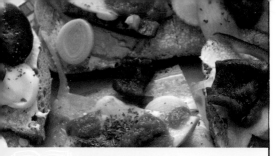

Recipe

Salmon and vegetable rainbow

Makes 6 to 8 servings.

Ingredients

80ml soy sauce
30ml rice wine vinegar
30ml vegetable oil
90g brown sugar
1 cherry-size piece of ginger,
    grated
2 garlic cloves, crushed
1 onion, chopped
1kg salmon or rainbow trout fillets
$1/2$ sweet red pepper cut into strips
1 carrot, cut into matchsticks
6 small yellow marrows, sliced
100g mangetout, halved
1 long aubergine, diced small

Preparation

Combine the first seven ingredients
    in a frying pan over medium
    heat. Cook until the onion is see-
    through, which should take
    about 3 minutes.
Add the fish and cook it for 3–5
    minutes. Turn the fish over, and
    cook it for another 3–5 minutes
    or until it is cooked through.
    Remove the fish to a serving
    dish and keep it warm.
Add the remaining ingredients to
    the frying pan. Cook over high
    heat just until vegetables are
    wilted. Put the vegetables on
    top of the salmon and serve.

Eating local produce

One of the principles of traditional diets, such as the Mediterranean, Asian or Latin American, is to eat locally grown vegetables that are in season. Then, the vegetables are richest in nutrients.

A mixture of vegetables

If you live in Central and South America, your diet might include okra, tomatillos and chillies, in addition to broccoli, spinach, aubergines and onions. In Asia, tiny aubergines, bamboo shoots, beans, various mushrooms, seaweeds and many different green vegetables might appear in your meals. Among the greens are bok choi, napa and flowering cabbages.

In the countries around the Mediterranean Sea, greens such as dandelion, mustard, rocket and nettles are sometimes featured in dishes.

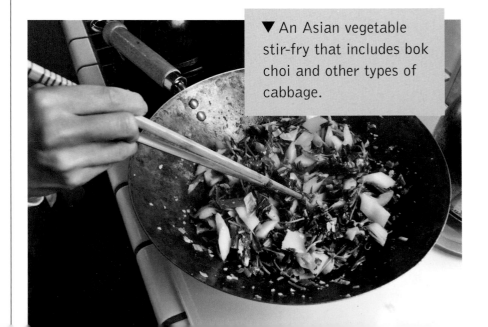

▼ An Asian vegetable stir-fry that includes bok choi and other types of cabbage.

Nutrition facts

Cooking vegetables

Quick-cooking methods – steaming, microwaving and stir-frying – are best for many vegetables. Cooked for too long, vegetables become mushy and unappealing, and lose many of their valuable nutrients.

When stir-frying, be sure to use a liquid vegetable oil, such as olive or rapeseed, to avoid adding unwanted saturated fat.

Baking vegetables such as potatoes, sweet potatoes and winter squashes in an oven keeps most of their flavours and nutrients. Grilled aubergine slices, mushrooms, red peppers, marrows and cauliflower can be enjoyed alone or served with meat or fish.

Vegetables as staples

In parts of the world, vegetables are a staple food – that is, the main source of nutrients and energy. In South America, Africa and India cassava is eaten widely. The roots are peeled, cooked and mashed. Taro, another root vegetable, is a staple in the tropics, and is used to make a thick food paste, poi, in Hawai'i. Yams are tubers similar to sweet potatoes. Many species of yam are eaten throughout Africa, Asia and South America.

In many part of Europe, the potato is a staple vegetable. It is eaten boiled, baked, sautéed and fried.

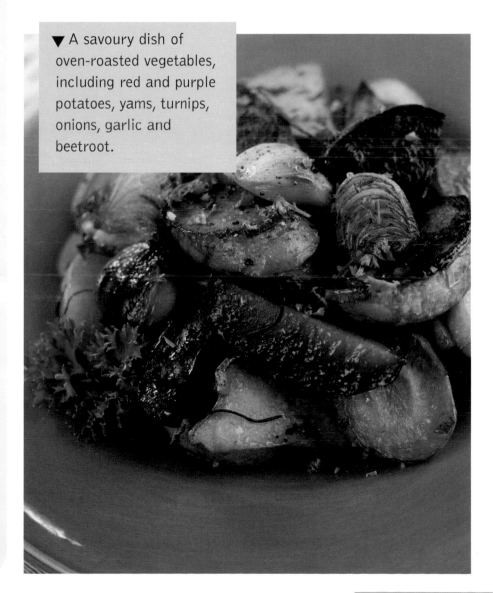

▼ A savoury dish of oven-roasted vegetables, including red and purple potatoes, yams, turnips, onions, garlic and beetroot.

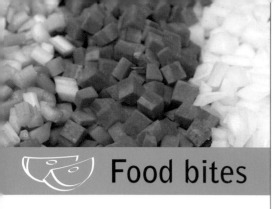

Food bites

Salsa for zest

Salsa is a spicy, tomato-based sauce. It is delicious with potatoes, eggs, rice, beans or pasta. It also makes a great low-fat dip. The tomatoes used for most salsas offer vitamin C, lycopene (a powerful antioxidant) and fibre. Other ingredients often include oil, vinegar, garlic, cumin, coriander leaves and onions.

Making meals

Any healthy food you eat provides better nutrients and replaces unhealthy food you might otherwise eat. Here are some more tasty and fun ways to eat vegetables.

Breakfast and lunch

To start the day, try mushrooms, onions or tomatoes in an omelette or with scrambled eggs. Potatoes can be eaten as hash browns. As a drink, try tomato or carrot juice. Cherry tomatoes go well with almost any dish.

At lunch, crisp, fresh vegetables go well with any main course, be it a sandwich, soup or pizza. A selection of carrots, celery, multicoloured peppers,

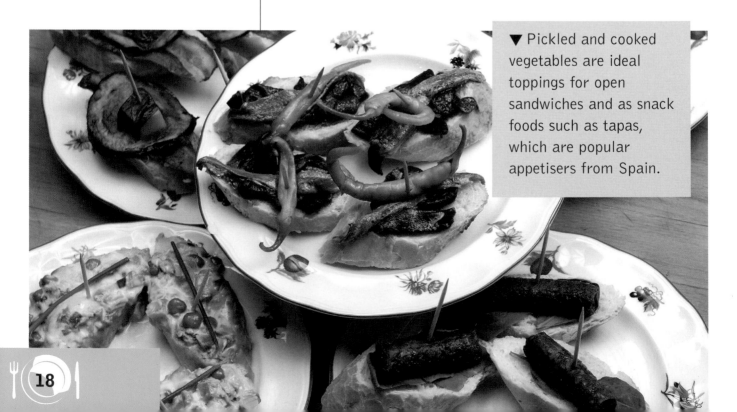

▼ Pickled and cooked vegetables are ideal toppings for open sandwiches and as snack foods such as tapas, which are popular appetisers from Spain.

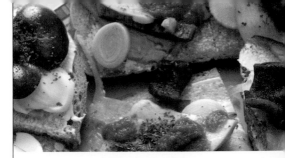

broccoli and cauliflower is perfect for your lunchbox. You can cut some of these vegetables into small pieces and keep them in the refrigerator for healthy snacks.

Leafy lettuces, spinach and herbs are great in salads, but also go well in sandwiches and wraps. You can also add some bean sprouts, strips of coloured peppers and cucumber slices. Any one of these ideas will easily add a serving of vegetables to your day.

Dinner

Vegetables are ideal for soups. Some soups, such as the Spanish soup gazpacho – made with cucumbers, green peppers, tomatoes and onions – are meant to be eaten cold. Almost any cooked vegetable can be eaten alongside meat or fish. Experiment with different kinds to suit your taste.

Try sprinkling chopped peppers or peas on rice or potatoes. Stir fry vegetables with small amounts of meat, fish or poultry to make an ideal quick dinner. Add grated carrots or courgettes to minced beef when making meatballs or to the dough for breads.

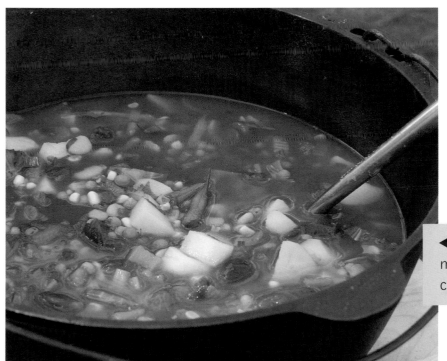

Recipe

Cheery sweet potato quickbread

Makes one loaf.
Ingredients
200g sugar
120ml rapeseed oil
1 medium sweet potato, grated (approx 300g)
3 eggs
240g flour
5ml baking powder
2.5ml baking soda
5ml cinnamon
2.5ml cardamom
100g dried cherries or cranberries
110g pecan nuts

Preparation
Preheat the oven to 100°C (Gas mark 4). In a large bowl, combine the ingredients in the order listed.
Turn the mixture into an oiled loaf pan. Bake the mixture for 50 minutes or until the bread looks done.
Cool the bread on wire racks and serve fresh.

◀ A hot, thick vegetable soup makes a satisfying meal for a cold winter's night.

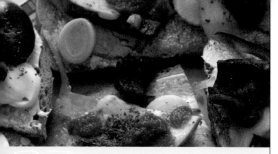

Recipe

Beany greeny pasta

Makes 8 servings.
Ingredients
280g uncooked macaroni
4 small heads baby bok choi or
    any dark, leafy green vegetable,
    cut into 3-cm lengths
3 400-g tins cannellini or any
    white beans, drained and rinsed
2 400-g tins diced tomatoes
2 garlic cloves, minced
2.5ml thyme
pepper, to taste
fresh grated parmesan cheese
    (optional: vegans can leave out)

Preparation
Cook the macaroni in boiling
    water. When it begins to soften –
    about 5 minutes – add the bok
    choi or other greens. Continue
    cooking until the macaroni is
    done, in about 3 more minutes.
Drain the macaroni and greens and
    return them to the pan. Add the
    beans, tomatoes, garlic, thyme
    and pepper, and stir to combine.
Cook until the mixture is heated
    through.
Serve with the cheese on the side.

As an alternative to baby bok choi,
    try spinach or Swiss chard. You
    might also add aubergines,
    courgettes and mushrooms.

Vegetarians and vegans

A vegetarian diet can include foods from all five of the food groups, as listed on page 6. If you are a vegan, your choices are limited to those of three groups – bread and other grain foods, fruits and vegetables, nuts and seeds – with some foods from the last group, fatty, sugary and salty foods. But you can still eat a varied, interesting and balanced diet.

Some of the websites listed on page 31 will give you ideas for vegetarian and vegan dishes and meals.

▼ A vegetable and tofu stir-fry is a nutritious vegetarian or vegan meal. Tofu is a protein-rich food made from soy milk.

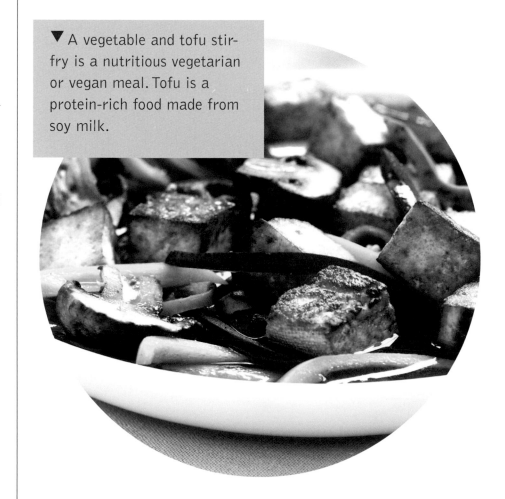

Vegetables with everything

One advantage of animal-based foods – meat, eggs, fish and dairy products – is that they give you all the different kinds of protein you need in one convenient package. Most vegetables contain very little protein, but nuts, seeds, pulses and grains can supply some. If you do not eat meat, you should eat vegetables with as wide a range of other plants foods as possible.

For soups and stews, mix vegetables with beans, lentils and grains such as barley. For salads, mix leafy green vegetables such as lettuce, spinach leaves and watercress with tomatoes, olives and walnuts. Root and tuber vegetables go well in savoury pies and pasties.

Back to basics

Remember to eat vegetables of different colours, and try to eat lots of fresh, raw vegetables. To keep all the goodness, try eating vegetables with the skin or peel on – see page 26 for information – and choose healthy cooking methods – see page 17. You can use sauces and herbs to add flavour and interest to many dishes.

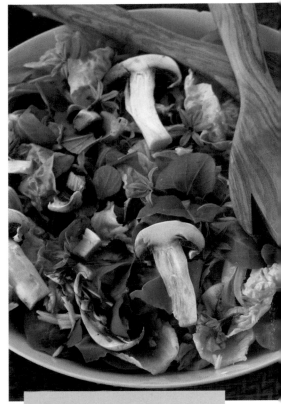

▲ Dress up your salads with mushrooms and fresh herbs, with edible flowers for added colour.

Nutrition facts

Getting all the minerals you need

Vegetable sources for nutrients found in animal foods:

calcium:	chickory, kale, broccoli, haricot beans, carrots, celery, watercress, spinach
copper:	sweet potatoes, broad beans, mushrooms
iron:	cashews, tomato juice, rice, tofu, lentils, chickpeas, spinach
phosphorus:	broad beans, kiwi fruit, spinach, asparagus, peppers, marrows
zinc:	Brussels sprouts, watercress, beetroot, parsnips, pumpkins, peppers

Digesting vegetables

Digestion is the process of breaking down everything you eat and drink to release the nutrients and to take them into your body. Vegetable food, being a mix of carbohydrates, proteins, minerals, vitamins and fibre, is broken down in many stages as it passes along your digestive system.

Digestion of vegetables starts in the mouth. With your teeth and tongue, you break food into tiny pieces. A watery liquid, saliva, is added to the food from glands in your mouth. Saliva contains chemicals called enzymes that attack carbohydrates, breaking them into simple sugars. These later get broken down further.

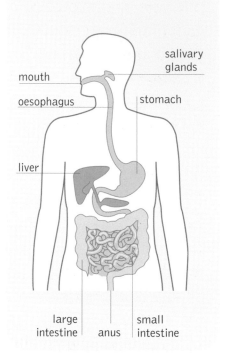

Health facts

The digestive system

salivary glands

mouth

oesophagus

stomach

liver

large intestine

anus

small intestine

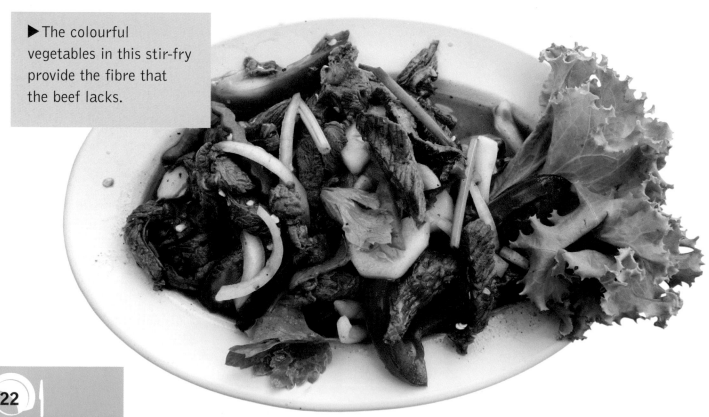

▶ The colourful vegetables in this stir-fry provide the fibre that the beef lacks.

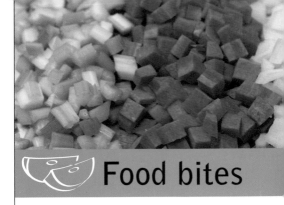

Down the tube

The partly digested food passes down your oesophagus to your stomach. There, many more enzymes are added. These start to break down proteins. Acid in your stomach kills any bacteria in the food and gets some minerals ready to pass into your blood system later on. Some water and sugars pass now into your blood.

Food moves from the stomach into your intestines. Lots more enzymes are added to the food. These complete the chemical breakdown of proteins and carbohydrates, and digest any fats.

The end products

During digestion, carbohydrates are broken down into the simple sugar glucose. Proteins become simpler chemicals known as amino acids. Fats are broken down into fatty acids and lipids. These all enter your blood system and are transported round your body. Along with them go all the minerals and vitamins and the rest of the water. Soluble and insoluble fibre pass through your digestive system without being broken down. They sweep away faeces, the waste products of digestion.

Food bites

Food allergies

Vegetables rarely cause food allergies, unlike foods such as nuts, shellfish and grains, which are known to cause problems. These unpleasant reactions to particular foods make you feel as if your body is being attacked by a virus or poison. Most allergic reactions to vegetables are mild, resulting in nothing worse than a rash or itching.

Nutrition facts

You need only small amounts of vitamins, but they are critical for good health.

name	benefits	found in
Vitamin A	healthy eyes, blood	vegetables and fruits, breakfast cereals, dairy products
B vitamins	prevent heart disease	many vegetables, dairy products, fish, eggs
Vitamin C	fights infections	vegetables and fruits (especially citrus)
Vitamin D	healthy bones	sunlight, dairy products, fortified cereals, fatty fish
Vitamin E	prevents cell damage	green leafy vegetables, grains, vegetable oils, nuts
Vitamin K	healthy blood, bones	dark green leafy vegetables, vegetable oils

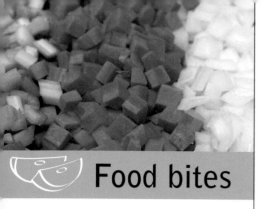

Food bites

Low energy

Vegetables are often counted as 'free food'. For many of them, you can eat as much as you want without putting on weight. Digesting them uses up almost all the kilocalories they contain. In fact, it takes more kilocalories to digest asparagus, beets, broccoli, green cabbage, carrots, cauliflower and celery than they offer.

Energy and body weight

Kilocalories – often shortened to kcal – are a measure of the energy in food. Vegetables do not have many kilocalories. A 100 gram portion of boiled potatoes contains only 80 kcal, and lettuce only 8 kcal, while 100 grams of fish fingers contain 178, cooked ham 269 and cheddar cheese 412. So you can eat lots of vegetables without taking in too much energy. Extra energy is stored in your body as fat.

The average child needs about 2,000 kilocalories a day. Young teenage girls need about 2,200 kcal and boys of the same age about 2,500 kcal a day. You need more kilocalories the more active you are. You get energy from food and drinks, as the list on page 25 shows.

Body Mass Index

To find your BMI number (see opposite), divide your height (in metres) by your weight (in kilograms). Divide the result by your weight again. The number should be near the average – the red line on each chart.

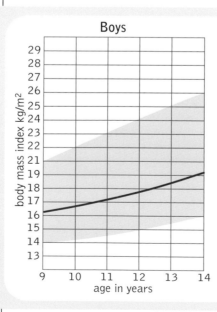

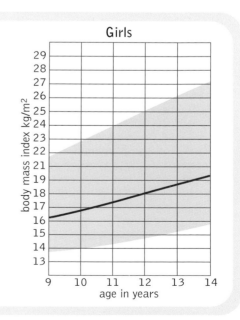

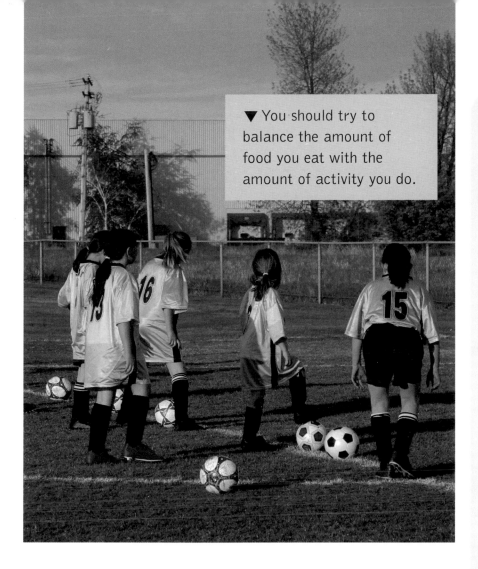

▼ You should try to balance the amount of food you eat with the amount of activity you do.

Balancing your energy

To stay fit and healthy, you need to balance the energy you take in with your needs. As a guide to whether you are in shape or not, some dieticians and doctors use your Body Mass Index (BMI). This a number that shows how your weight (mass) compares to your height. If your number is within that of much of the population, you are in the healthy range. It shows you are getting a good balance of food and exercise.

A high BMI can sometimes result if you have lots of muscle, or if your body is preparing for a growth spurt. But if your diet needs improvement, try some of the ideas in this book. Plain fresh vegetables are one food you can eat as much of as you want without fear of putting on too much weight.

Nutrition facts

A day's energy intake

kcal	meals
	breakfast
221	2-egg mushroom and spinach omelette
136	2 slices rye toast
102	1 glass semi-skimmed milk
	lunch
278	chicken breast sandwich on wholemeal bread, with cucumber and sprouts
112	1 oatmeal biscuit
69	1 orange
	snack
223	celery and carrot slices with hummus
177	1 glass tomato juice
	dinner
72	small bowl of vegetable soup
291	small grilled steak
27	1 cup steamed broccoli
145	1 baked potato
80	leafy, green salad with oil and vinegar
125	1 scoop ice cream
2,058	GRAND TOTAL

Nutrition facts

Skins and peels

Vegetables should be washed in clear, cool water to remove any dirt, pesticides and microorganisms, which can cause food-poisoning. Even pre-washed salad greens should be washed again before you eat them. The outer leaves of vegetables such as cabbage should be removed and thrown away.

Vegetable skins and peels generally contain nutrients and fibre, so eat them when they can be cleaned. The skins of potatoes, beets and cucumbers can be gently scrubbed with a brush.

Shopping and storing

You can buy most vegetables fresh at local shops, market stalls or in supermarkets. Choose produce that is brightly coloured and free of blemishes. Leaf vegetables should be crisp. Do not buy bruised vegetables as they will spoil quickly. Look for vegetables that are in season, and only buy as much as you will eat within a few days.

Fresh or prepared

In shops and supermarkets, green leafy vegetables may be prepacked in see-through bags. Many vegetables come frozen, pickled or dried, in packs or in tins. Vegetable juices come in bottles or cartons. Look at labels on the packaging for details of how long the food will stay fresh, how to store it and how to cook it.

▶In market stalls, vegetables are on display. If you want to choose your own vegetables, ask the salesperson first if you can do this.

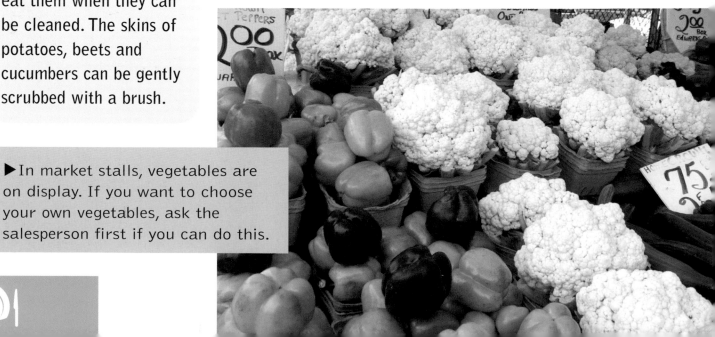

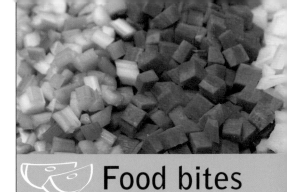

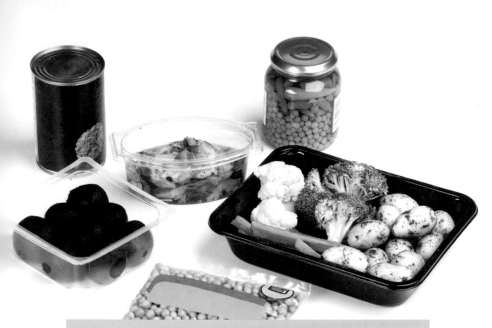

▲ In shops and supermarkets, vegetables are sold fresh, in tins, jars, plastic bags and cartons.

Frozen or tinned vegetables are processed within hours of harvesting so are very nutritious. In general, though, fresh vegetables are richer in nutrients than frozen, and frozen are more nutritious than tinned.

Some supermarkets sell ready-made vegetable dishes that can be put in a microwave and heated in minutes. The more ready-made or prepared a food is, the more unwanted salt, flavourings and colours have been added to it. These foods should not be a major part of your diet.

Look at the label

Check the list of ingredients and nutritional information on packaged foods. Should you be a vegetarian or vegan, or if you have a food allergy, look out for relevant details. Reading the labels on packages will also help you choose vegetable dishes that are high in protein, fibre, minerals and vitamins, and low in saturated fat and salt. The labels will also give you details of the kilocalories in the food.

Food bites

Storing

Do not wash vegetables until you are ready to eat them. Store root vegetables in a cool, dark place. Other vegetables should be kept in a crisper drawer in the refrigerator. Be sure that red meats, fish and poultry are stored below other foods so their juices cannot drop on food that you will be eating raw. Mouldy or slimy vegetables should be thrown away.

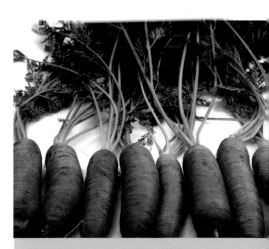

▲ Vegetables like carrots stay fresher if the tops are left on.

Cooking safety

Here are some rules you should follow when cooking and following recipes.

- ask an adult for permission to cook and for help in handling anything sharp or hot
- wash your hands before you begin
- after handling raw meat, wash your hands, cooking tools and surfaces with hot, soapy water
- wash fruits and vegetables before using
- use pot holders or oven gloves when handling something hot
- keep pot handles turned towards the back of the stove
- open pan lids away from you to avoid burning your face with steam
- avoid loose long sleeves, or roll them up
- keep your fingers and hair out of the way when using appliances
- never plug in appliances with wet hands

Projects

Here are some ideas for things you can do related to vegetables and diet. Discover the variety of vegetables that is available. Record what you are eating now and see how you can introduce more vegetables into a balanced diet.

 ## Action 1

Supermarket detective

- How many different kinds of fresh vegetables can you find in your local supermarket? Are any of them organically grown (see page 12)?
- Write down their names, then group them according to the parts of the plants they are – leaves, stems, roots, tubers and so on. Next, group the vegetables according to their colour.
- Look at the labels to find which countries the vegetables came from. Do some countries seem to produce more vegetables than others and, if so, of which types of vegetables?
- Take a look at the tinned, frozen and dried food sections in the supermarket. How many different kinds of vegetables can you find?
- Look at the juice section. How many kinds of vegetable juices are there? Is this more or less what you expected?

Action 2

Food tracking

Make a chart like the one shown below. For five days, every time you eat a serving of vegetables, put a tick into the appropriate box or boxes.

If you eat a vegetable of an unusual colour, record its details in the bottom box, for example purple potatoes, orange beets or black carrots.

At the end of the five days, count the number of servings for each day. Write these totals in the bottom row. Now, add up how many vegetables of different colours you ate during the period. Write these totals in the right-hand column.

VEGETABLE COLOURS	Monday	Tuesday	Wednesday	Thursday	Friday	Total colours
red						
orange						
yellow						
green						
blue purple						
white						
unusual colours						
TOTAL SERVINGS						

- On how many days did you eat at least five servings?
- On how many days did you eat vegetables of every colour?
- Which colour did you eat the most often?

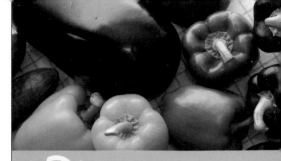

Action 3

Something new

Buy an unfamiliar vegetable. Search on the Internet and find an easy recipe for it. Try cooking the vegetable (ask for help if you need it). Make a survey of your family. Who liked the new vegetable? Who did not? Would you cook it and eat it again?

See what you can learn about the part of the world the vegetable comes from and the people who eat it regularly.

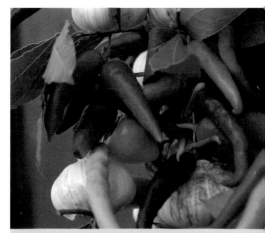

▲ Fresh chillies and garlic.

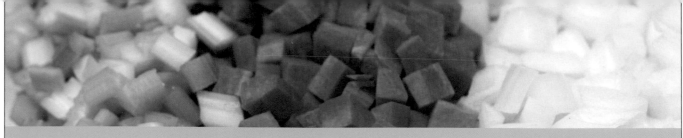

Glossary

CARBOHYDRATES
One of the three main nutrients in food. They are made of sugar molecules and mostly provide energy.

DIET
The food and drink that a person eats.

ENZYMES
Substances that help digestion and other chemical processes.

FATS
One of the three main nutrients in food. They are made of fatty acids and glycerol and mostly provide an energy store.

FERTILISERS
Substances put on the ground to enrich the soil.

GRAINS
The seeds of grass plants.

INGREDIENTS
Items of food used to make a dish.

KILOCALORIES (kcal)
The units used to measure the energy in foods and drinks.

MINERALS
Nutrients needed for health. They include iron, calcium, sodium and zinc.

NUTRIENTS
Materials the body needs but cannot make itself. Foods rich in nutrients are said to be nutritious.

PESTICIDES
Chemicals put on plants and soil to kill pests and germs.

POULTRY
Birds kept for meat and eggs, in particular chickens, turkeys and ducks.

PROTEINS
One of the three main nutrients in food. They are made of amino acids and mostly provide building materials for the body.

PULSES
Dried beans, peas and lentils.

RED MEAT
Meat rich in blood, such as beef, lamb, veal and pork.

ROOT
An underground part of a plant that takes up water and minerals from the soil.

SATURATED FATS
Fats found mainly in animal foods. Eating too much saturated fat can raise levels of cholesterol in the blood, increasing the risk of heart disease.

STEM
A part of a plant, usually above ground, from which grow roots and shoots with leaves and flowers.

TUBER
A swollen part of some plants, usually underground, that can grow both stems and roots.

VITAMINS
Nutrients needed for health, fitness and body processes.

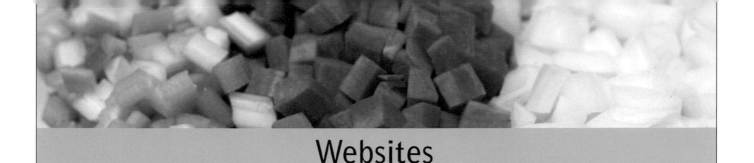

Websites

Here is a selection of websites that give information and activities about food, diet, health and fitness. Some deal only with vegetables. Others are more general but include vegetables.

http://www.5aday.nhs.uk/
Information from the National Health Service on eating vegetables and fruits.

http://www.thinkvegetables.co.uk/
All about vegetables: nutrition, what is in season, and growers.

http://www.eatwell.gov.uk/healthydiet/
    nutritionessentials/fruitandveg/
Nutritional information from the Food Standards Agency, focusing on vegetables and fruits.

http://www.pickyourownfarms.org.uk
Find a farm near you where you can pick your own vegetables.

http://vickids.tamu.edu/nutrition/index.
    html
Vegetable and fruit information, tips and games for kids.

http://www.vegsoc.org/info/foodfacts.
    html
Information about a vegetarian diet.

http://foodsubs.com/FGVegetables.html
Extensive information on different kinds of vegetables, including photographs and cooking tips.

http://www.passionateaboutfood.net/
    healthy.php
A wide variety of information about food, with recipes and advice.

http://library.thinkquest.org/4485/
    frames.htm
Gives information and advice on food and diet, focusing on fast foods.

http://www.foodafactoflife.org.uk/
Educational material about food, diet and nutrients.

Index